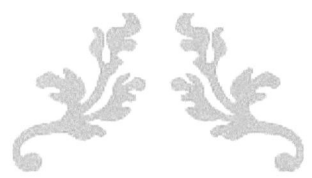

SECRETS FOR HEALTHY LIVING

How to Change Your Life by Eating Right

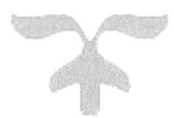

Chinele Prince

This book belongs to

_____

_____

_____

"Information is knowledge." -Albert Einstein

Acknowledgments

This book is dedicated to the Holy Spirit, my constant Friend and Helper whose invaluable love, support and guidance has made my life meaningful. I would like to thank those who have been there for me over the years : my beloved husband Pastor CNS Prince, my amazing daughter and gift from God, Sharon Chimamanda, my siblings, the wonderful Women of Asset group for providing a prayer cover for me, my weekly prayer partners Charity Chujor and Fidel for persistently praying for my family and ministry, my Mother-in-law who loves me dearly, and Pastor Sam

King who was always helpful during

my master's program.

I thank everyone who has been kind

to me in my journey through life. I love

you all!

*"The road to life is a
disciplined life;
ignore correction
and you're lost for
good"*

(Proverbs 10:17, MSG).

CONTENTS

Introduction

Quinoa

Raspberries

Spinach

Walnuts

Acai

Banana

Avocado

Watercress

Chia Seeds

Coconut

Apples

Superfood drinks

Flat belly juice

Hot lemon tea

x

INTRODUCTION

This book is about implementing a healthy diet and promoting weight loss through proper eating habits. It shows how preparing a nutritious diet, eating healthy and cultivating a healthy lifestyle can be so easy and fun. I can assure you that the healthy recipes presented in this book will work for anybody and help you shed weight every single week without much stress. Through discipline and commitment, you will be able to incorporate natural foods and drinks into your regular diet thus investing in your health. Even if you struggle with food cravings or find it difficult to motivate yourself to exercise, the information in this book will help you improve your emotional and physical health, lose weight, prevent illness, and enhance your natural beauty and look amazing. I am a testimony to this because soon after I began the quest to transform my health, I found that weight loss and wellness aren't far-fetched. You can achieve both if you utilize the right methods.

The question you must ask yourself is, "how much do I want to change my eating habits?" "What sacrifices are my

willing to make to achieve my goal?"
Believe in yourself and use the power
of positive thinking to encourage
yourself. The choice is yours. You must
be focused and follow through on
your tasks as you commit to your
desire weight loss goal and to eating
healthy. Each day take actions that
bring you closer to the way you want
to look and feel. Do yourself a fav or
and be bold about your decision
because thereafter, you will enjoy a
very vibrant life full of energy and joy.
Most people think that being
overweight is merely the consequence

of eating too much and not exercising well enough. However, certain psychological factors also play a role in this. For example, people who are impulsive eaters are more likely to be overweight than conscientious eaters. Also, people who do not sleep enough or who are stressed will likely gain more weight than those who exercise and are relaxed. Nonetheless, change always begins in the mind. It is a decision you must make only if you are willing to pay the price for the change you desire. Making long-term changes

in your daily eating and exercise

habits will deliver long-lasting results.

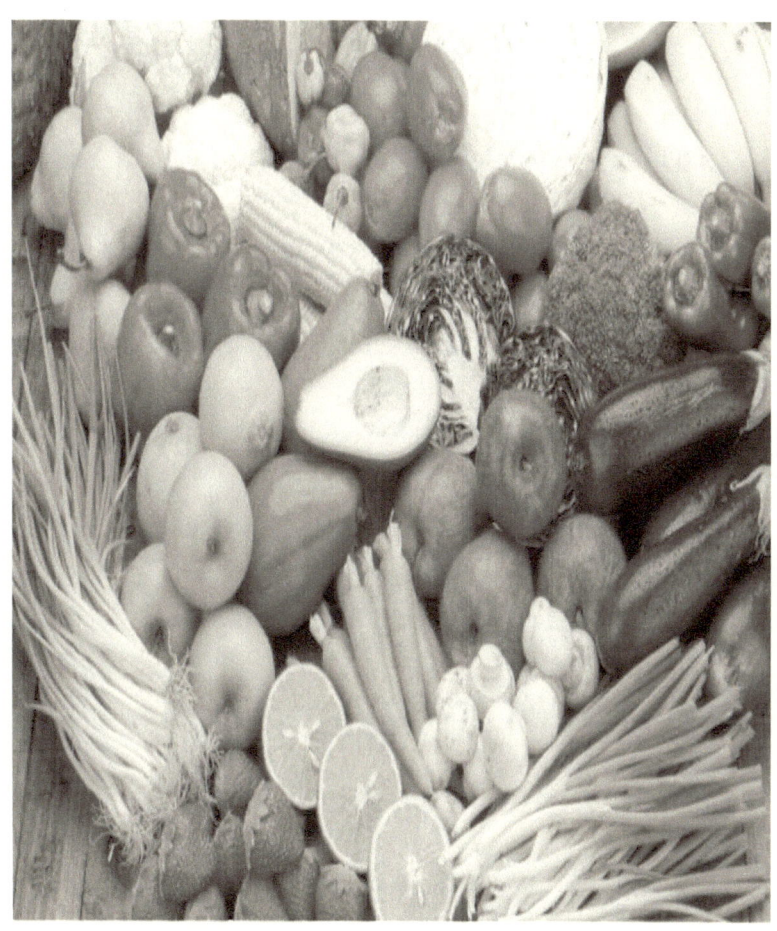

Chapter one

Have a Plan

My journey to embracing natural foods as a health remedy began rather fortuitously. I was diagnosed with type two diabetes while in my early forties. I was staggered because none of my parents had diabetes. My father loved to feast on sugar. He indulged a lot of starchy foods too. He liv ed to be 83 and he never had diabetes, neither was he obese. I guess his metabolism was great! On the other hand, I avoided eating sugar. I had always eaten healthy, but the doctor said my cortisol was very high and the reason was I'd been suffering from lack of sleep. I started having chronic fatigue, lower back pain, body aches, and blurry vision. I inadvertently, began to gain so much weight. Then, one night on my way home from work, I fell so sick I had to go to the emergency room. I had almost fainted at work. I was having chronic fatigue, increased thirst as well as frequent urination. I was told I had to pay a consultation fee of five hundred dollars and then the final bill would be sent to me after the doctor had attended to me. I didn't have medical insurance at the time because we had just mov ed from Maryland to Texas. It was a difficult decision to make but I decided not to see the doctor. I thought the charges were rather expensive and so I walked away. I was conflicted about paying five hundred dollars just to be reminded what I needed to do—to make better choices concerning the food I ate and to lose weight. I knew I was taking a risk, but I felt at peace with my decision. I had to take drastic steps to overcome my health challenge. That night I prayed and told my prayer partners to agree with me about my health. I began researching natural ways to control blood sugar and the best foods to eat in order to lose weight. I studied how to increase my metabolism and boost my energy level. Over a period of three months, I gradually started seeing results. The back pain left. My mental clarity improv ed. My skin began to glow, revealing a beautiful complexion. I felt energized and I was finally losing weight! People started asking me the secret to my weight loss and I decided to write a book so that others could benefit from the story of

my transformation.

I lost 40 pounds in 3 months! I realized

that my body could be younger and

fresher than my actual age depending

on my diet, lifestyle choices, and

physical activities. I will go into details

about my methods in this book. All you

need is the discipline to focus on

making better food choices. I

encourage you to eat whole grains,

lean meats, vegetables, and fresh fruits

with lots of antioxidants. This is the best

way to achieve optimum wellness.

Eventually, you will love yourself more and celebrate your weight loss success. I had always wanted to become an author since I was a young girl, but I wasn't sure of the exact path to take or the literary genre to focus on. I always enjoyed reading and despite the wealth of knowledge I got, putting my thoughts on paper prov ed to be a challenge. However, I set a goal to write my first book and I am thrilled to have accomplished it. The Scripture tells us that all things work together for good to those that love the Lord and are called according to His

purpose (Rom 8:28).

I wrote this nutritional book as I

researched about divine health and I

truly believe it is part of my calling to help

people incorporate healthy eating

habits into their diet. My goal is to give

sound and effective information on what

is best to eat and drink for optimum

health. This book will be a guide to

encouraging positive, healthy eating

habits. Remember, you have control

over what you put in your body, and the

better you take care of your body the

healthier you will be. I care

about my body and my state of mind because I have only one body.

Having knowledge of how your body works, and planning what best fits your personality will make you enjoy a happy and healthy lifestyle.

Set a goal for your transformation and ask yourself what you want to achieve at the end of it all. This will set you up for success because you have made the first step that will act like a foundation for everything going forward. It might seem like a difficult journey, but if you set your mind to enjoy the process rather than enduring it, then your confidence to complete the journey will increase as you begin to see encouraging results. The major goals you can set include eating healthier, achieve weight loss, burning excess belly fat, increasing your metabolism, strengthening your muscles, looking more beautiful, and reducing high blood pressure. Thereafter, establish strategies that will enable you accomplish these goals. Develop a weekly schedule that focuses on the change you desire. Encourage yourself by focusing on the benefits of being healthy. Visualize what you would look like after your radical transformation. This will motivate you to work harder. Be diligent and don't give up even if you do not see immediate changes. I saw my first results after the third week. Having a huge meal isn't the same as having a good meal. A huge meal focuses on just getting full whereas a good meal focuses on not just how healthy it is but on the right amount to eat. Set a date to prep your meal and a time for your physical workout. For example, boil eggs for a grab-and-go snack, together with some cucumber,

or almonds and put them in a
Ziploc bag.

I encourage you to find a partner or be
around people who share your goals. It
encourages accountability. It could be
your friends, spouse, children, neighbor,
co-workers or bible study group. Be
deliberate about knowing the food
you want to eat. Be mindful of what
you put into your mouth. Don't wait too
long to put healthy food or drink into
your system. We often starve ourselves
in the name of watching our weight
instead of eating what is healthy at the
appropriate time. For

example, Berries are a good snack for breakfast, nuts are an enjoyable snack for lunch while cucumbers are an extremely good snack to have after dinner. It is advisable to turn off the television or put down your phone when eating because it will prompt you to eat less. Try to eat slowly and enjoy your meal.

There are two main ways to lose weight and maintain adequate weight. First, eat a low-calorie diet that requires little exercise. Second, eat a high-calorie diet that will hav e to make you implement more exercises in your plan.

Choose the option that works best

for you.

My personal adv ice is to hav e balance.

That means to always eat plant-based

foods with low carbs, make sure to drink

plenty of water, and let the

beverages you drink be low calorie

drinks. Always remember to

exercise moderately but regularly.

CHAPTER 2

Health Goals

Success is as simple as setting sustainable goals if you make them SMART. S.M.A.R.T. is an acronym that stands for specific, measurable, attainable, realistic and timely. SMART goals are helpful for keeping us focused on doing the things that bring us closer to accomplishing our goals. An example of a Specific goal is to join a health club and work out three days a week. You can Measure your progress when you stay on track yet reach your target date. You can Attain your goals when you plan your steps wisely and establish a time frame that allows you to carry out those steps. Be accountable to yourself and your support system of friends and family to accomplish your SMART goals. Your Realistic goal should be tailored to your personality type if you truly believe that it can be accomplished.

A goal should be grounded within a time frame. If you want to lose 10 pounds, set a deadline for accomplishing it. If you anchor it within a timeframe, for instance, "by May 7," or "before my wedding anniversary," then you hav e set your

unconscious mind into motion to

begin working on the goal.

T̲ also stands for tangible. It's a goal you

can experience with one of the senses;

taste, touch, smell, sight or hearing.

When your goal is tangible you have a

better chance of making it specific

and measurable and thus attainable.

Practice self-care

Self-care is about taking care of

yourself to improv e your emotional,

physical and mental well-being. It

includes getting enough sleep,

relaxation, and managing your stress to

improv e your health. It is ideal to do a 4-week weight-loss plan that caters to your personality. It doesn't hurt to go for a massage which can alleviate sore muscles and pain. Massages help in stimulating proper blood circulation and are a great stress reliever. Similarly, enjoy yourself and do sauna or heat therapy to purify your mind and body. It will help you lower blood pressure, lose weight, reduce stress and make you glow. But remember to drink water before and after the sauna. Affirm and celebrate yourself. Speak positively to yourself each day.

I say to myself:

I am blessed

I am wise

I am a good distributor

I am born for greatness

I am a seed of

Abraham I am favored

I am chosen

I am redeemed

I am honorable

I am different

I am important I

am prosperous I

am successful I

am beautiful

I am accepted

I am confident

I am content

I am healed

I am deeply loved

I love God

I love myself! Victory

is my lifestyle

Thank you, Jesus! Hallelujah!

Why Choose Healthy Lifestyle Goals?

I wanted my skin to look better

and fresher.

I wanted to be able to put my body

in a position to become even fitter

overall.

I wanted to be healthy enough and become an excellent example to my peers.

I wanted to discipline myself to learn more about nutrition and health. I started eating my food slowly which helped me lose weight and I was enjoying my food a lot more. Eating slowly reduces stress and leads to better digestion.

I began studying herbs, spices, and foods that helped to produce a healthier lifestyle.

I also started to detox my body to increase my energy level, lower my body fat and remove harmful toxins. People started to notice the difference in my body, and they were impressed with the results. They wanted the same changes. I was able to accomplish more work towards my career and goals in a day because of my new healthy lifestyle. I created a detox and healthy meal choice program that shows how to naturally detoxify the body to increase energy levels, remove harmful toxins from the body and increase fat loss.

Finally, one thing that propelled me is that lifestyle change is better than being on prescription drugs.

Successful Weight-Loss Tips

• Drink purified water

• Drink lemon and ginger water

• Drink aloe-v era and cranberry

• Cut your calories and control your meal portions

• Snack on seeds and nuts such as almonds and walnuts

Eat more salads and vegetables like spinach, bitter leaf, peppermint leaf

Eat fruits like cucumber, grapefruit, berries, and avocado

- Add coconut oil to your diet

- Add apple cider vinegar to your diet

and drink

- Exercise regularly

- Sleep adequately.

Chapter 3

Lifestyle Goals for Healthy Living

Sleep

For me, sleeping at night has always been more of a luxury than a necessity. In the past I didn't sleep as much as I should have because I was more of a night person. But as I got older, I realized that the quantity and quality of sleep you have is a predictor of your energy and success. In order to establish better sleeping habits, make sure your room is dark. Invest in bedding that will make you comfortable. Use essential oils such as lavender and chamomile to create a calming atmosphere. I urge you to sleep and have adequate rest daily. Sleep affects the hormones that regulate appetite and metabolism and when the hormones are out of balance, there is an increase in appetite followed by an elevated craving for sugar and starchy foods like pasta and bread. People with the best health and longevity get at least 7 to 8 hours of sleep daily. Quality sleep should be like nourishment because it's the time our body works with the nutrients it received during the day which makes the body repair and recover during the night. Therefore, give yourself permission to sleep. One of the ways to sleep better is to try not to drink after night shower. The best tea to drink at night is Chamomile tea, lavender tea or passionflower tea which take away stress and make you sleep peacefully. Spray some lavender on yourself or in your room. Do some aromatherapy.

Aromatherapy: This is a holistic healing treatment that uses natural plant extracts to promote health and well-being. It's important to try to practice aromatherapy at least twice a week. It enhances both physical and emotional health. It could be as simple as having a hot bath which is an excellent way to reduce stress, care for the skin, release toxins from the body, sooth muscles, and detox by opening the pores. Add good essential oils and Epsom salt to warm water and soak yourself for about 30 minutes. This will help reduce muscle soreness, alleviates pain in the body and allow you to sleep deeply. You can put a few drops of essential oil (lavender, chamomile, rosemary, sandalwood) in your humidifier or diffuser in your room and certainly, you will enjoy a peaceful sleep. You can sprinkle a few drops of lavender or chamomile essential oils on your pillow to help alleviates insomnia. I like lavender, frankincense, and peppermint. The aroma is pleasant, and it brings a sense of calm and relaxation as well.

Benefits of Aromatherapy:

• It manages pain

- It improv es sleep quality

- It reduces stress and anxiety

- It soothes sore joints

- It treats headaches and migraines

- It alleviates the side effects

of chemotherapy

- It fights bacteria, virus, or fungus

- It improves digestion

- It relieves diarrhea

- It boosts immunity

Get regular physical activity: Aim for

30-60 minutes of physical activity daily.

Stress can cause anxiety, depression,

confusion, and difficulty concentrating.

Eventually, it can disrupt your daily

activities. Therefore, do not stress yourself. Exercise is a stress reliever and helps in detoxification. It also improv es heart function and flexibility of joints. When it comes to exercise, little but often is the golden rule.

Organic Foods: Eat more plant-based foods such as peas, beans and nuts. These are good sources of plant proteins. Salads are one of the keys to eating a healthy diet. It is vital to eat at least one serving of salad a day. Eat more whole grains daily such as oatmeal.

Choose healthy fats: Eat at least 1 serving of nuts daily (2 tablespoons of peanut or almond butter). Eat foods high in 3 fatty acids daily such as flax meal, walnuts, almonds, and avocado.

Maintain a healthy weight: A BMI of less than 25 is ideal. Know and follow a healthy nutritional guideline. Try to have the normal weight for your body. Make sure to track your progress.

Be Joyful: Be cheerful always and display a positive attitude often. Choose to see the brighter side of life. Try to write a grateful journal in which you detail what you have and why you are grateful for them. Laugh a lot and practice smiling. This works like magic.

Relationships: Spend quality time with family or friends who really love you. Supportive and beneficial relationships build strong hearts and happy minds. Share kindness with someone daily. Try life coaching with me or any other person that helps you stay inspired. Join a bible study group, or a prayer group where you can feel accepted and find support and encouragement. I would recommend the Midnight Commanders Prayer Network (midnightcommanders.com), a prayer support group that caters to

the spiritual needs of people.

Renewal: Take time daily for spiritual

renewal: Plan a quiet time each day

to read, pray, meditate, and seek

spiritual renewal. Try to set aside one

day in a week to rest and reflect.

Fasting is very healthy. It is a rest from

food. It helps our body detoxify and

rejuvenate. It will help prevent health

problems. It gives mental clarity and

spiritual alertness.

Be prosperous: Do not liv e above your

means. Try to save no matter how

much you earn. Scripture tells us to owe

no man anything except to lov e one

another (Rom 13:8). Ramsey (2013)

says, "No one is born with the

knowledge of how to handle money"

(p.75). Thus, the ability to manage

money wisely is a learned behavior.

Choose giving over receiving.

Eat Right Everyday

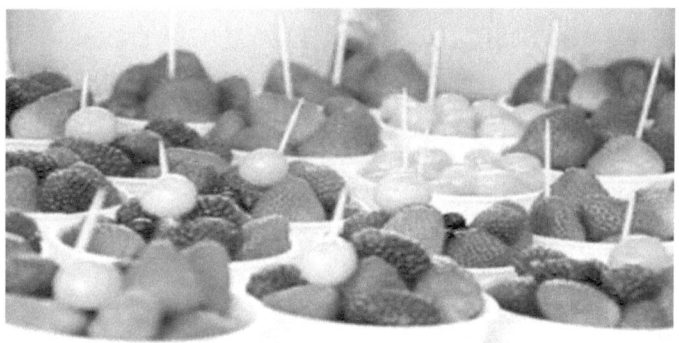

Eating the right foods will make you feel

healthy and the nutrients you gain will

help your body's immune system fight

diseases rather than relying on medication to combat health issues. Eating right makes you proactively healthy. Similarly, nutrients provide energy that makes you feel good physically. Each time you eat, have a mix of protein, fats, and little carbs. It is healthy for instance, to dip cucumber in peanut butter or almond butter. The key to losing weight is having a healthy metabolism. Good metabolism is the process that turns food into fuel. Eat one-ingredient foods that are unprocessed, are in their natural form, and are easily digestible, such as garden egg, carrot, apple, blueberry, beans, coconut, and avocados. Protein is very good at making your metabolism work and helping your body to repair itself. The healthy fats you should eat are olive oil, coconut oil, avocado, nuts, and seeds. The golden hour to eat or drink which will promote burning fat for weight loss is at least 45 minutes before going to bed. Try to eat a snack in between meals. So, if you eat lunch at noon and dinner at eight, you can have a mini meal in between and then try not to eat later.

Each time you eat, have a combination of proteins, fats, and carbs in order to prevent your blood sugar from spiking. Try drinking warm Chamomile tea or lavender tea at night. It will make you sleep better and feel better. Cucumber is a healthy choice if you have sudden food cravings. Apple is great but it is better with peanut butter, almond butter, or cottage cheese which will make you feel full. Focus on anything high on antioxidants, like pomegranates or berries to neutralize the free radicals in your body. Free radicals are a stressor to the body. Matcha tea is a powdered and processed green tea leaf. It has more antioxidants than coffee and it promotes focus and alertness. So, the best time to drink matcha tea is in the morning or early afternoon, due to the caffeine content.

Here are Foods that Fight Pain

✓Cherries help reduce
tissue inflammation

✓Green tea helps reduce inflammation

✓Olive oil helps reduce the risk of
stroke and cancer

✓Turmeric helps to fight
chronic inflammation

Fiber is the secret

Fibers are mostly found in oats, quinoa, almonds, chia seeds, beans, and raspberries. A high-fiber diet helps reduce the risk of obesity, heart disease, and diabetes. Fiber is an important nutrient that may promote weight loss, lower blood sugar levels and fight constipation. Fiber helps to keep your stomach fuller longer, so that you eat less during the day thereby maintaining your weight. It also helps to slow digestion. Good sources of fiber are bran, beans, whole grain, berries, avocados, green peas, nuts, sweet potatoes, brussels sprout, squash, and deep green leafy vegetables. It can reduce the risk of high blood pressure and heart attack. Therefore, fiber is essential because it will help your digestion and decrease carbohydrates in your food.

RIGHT HYDRATION

Water is the most natural healthy drink to consume. Water is said to comprise from 75% body weight in infants to 55% in the elderly. It helps you live cleaner because it cleanses your system. It serves as a lubricant in your joints and maintains body temperature. Water makes up much of our body weight. When we drink water in the morning, it increases our metabolism, that is, the rate at which our body burns calories. Water also helps us to hydrate when we sleep at night. Everyone of us needs about 8 glasses of water daily even though we will have to pee about 6 cups of it. Consequently, the more water we drink, the more we lose weight. Always have your water on the go since it's easy to get dehydrated. Dehydration is the cause of sagging energy, sore muscles, and cramping. The ideal thing to do is to drink more water in the morning and less at night in order to have a restful sleep. My research shows that drinking lemon water makes you lose pounds by causing you to pee more often. Therefore, it is not advisable to drink lemon water at night if you want to sleep without waking up to pee. But chamomile tea helps to calm anxiety and makes you sleep better.

Part of my secrets for healthy living was drinking lots of water throughout the day. My health started improving and I burned more calories. In the next chapter, I will tell you different infused water recipes for healthy balanced living. You will be drinking a lot of different flavored water made by you.

Drinking tea

Tea is a beverage that keeps you hydrated while you lose weight. Herbal tea has antioxidant and anti-inflammatory properties which strengthens digestion and boosts the immune system like turmeric tea.

Turmeric tea

1 teaspoon of turmeric

1 teaspoon of ginger

A dash of black pepper/cayenne pepper

1 teaspoon of natural honey

Boil 2 cups of water

Add all the ingredients and simmer

for 3 minutes. Strain in a cup and add

natural honey. You can also add

almond milk or coconut milk.

Green tea

This is one of the most popular herbal

teas due to its reputed health

benefits, such as weight loss, and

reduced stress. It promotes relaxation

and encourages mental clarity.

Peppermint tea

Peppermint tea reduces the feeling

of being full and can reduce

inflammation that causes bloating. It can help treat the feelings of nausea and prevents vomiting. It can lower your overall body temperature. Peppermint can relieve discomfort of the digestive tract. It can reduce stress and increase your overall wellbeing.

Matcha tea

Matcha tea is a natural laxative that can push toxins out of your system. It is rich in fiber, chlorophyll, and vitamins. It boosts your metabolism and lowers cholesterol. It has more antioxidant level than coffee and is stronger than green tea. Matcha strengthens

mood and aids in concentration.

Ingredients

I tablespoon of matcha

tea 3 slices of cucumber 2

slices of lemon

Add warm water, whisk and drink.

Passionflower Tea

Passionflower tea can relieve anxiety

and improv e sleep. For example, a

study found that drinking

passionflower tea can improv e sleep

quality. So, try to take it when you are

stress and you need to sleep.

Ginger tea

Ginger tea is a spicy and flavorful drink that packs a punch of healthy, disease-fighting antioxidants. It helps fight inflammation and stimulates the immune system. Ginger is effective at relieving nausea, especially in early pregnancy, although it may also relieve nausea caused by cancer treatments and motion sickness. I used to have stomach ulcers and ginger played a big part in my recovery. Ginger helps prevents stomach ulcers and relieve indigestion or constipation. Ginger may also help relieve dysmenorrhea or period pain. Several studies have found that ginger capsules reduce pain associated with menstruation. In fact, studies have found ginger to be as effective as non-steroidal anti-inflammatory drugs (NSAIDs) like ibuprofen at relieving period pain. Ginger offers health benefits for people with diabetes, though the evidence has not been consistent. Ginger tea is best known as a remedy for nausea and digestion.

DETOXIFICATION

The liver is the major organ for detoxification. The liver is vital for removing toxins. By detoxifying the body, we return balance to our body systems. This helps regulate our weight. The kidney plays a role in detox; thus, we need to drink a lot of water and eat plenty of fruits which have high water content to enable our kidney to remove waste products. Drink water If you are tired, have poor concentration, headache, dry lips, and dry skin.

Dandelion root tea can detox your system. It can provide liver decongestion by stimulating bile. It also can also help alleviate liver inflammation.

Honey Drink with Ginger and Lemon

This drink is a favorite not just for detox but also for managing an upset stomach. This drink will make you lose weight, stay focused and be energized.

Lemons: they are natural immunity boosters. They are packed with high levels of Vitamin C with other vitamins and minerals, calcium, magnesium, and can be used as natural cleansers. Lemon boasts antiviral and antibacterial abilities. Lemon contains flavonoids that help with the regulation of cholesterol and fatty acid. It even improv es your skin's general health. Because once everything is working properly on the inside, it accentuates a natural glow on your skin.

The Best Natural Laxative!

Ingredients

Dates

Prunes

Water

Bring the water to a boil, then add

chopped dates and prunes and

simmer the mixture for 10-15 minutes.

Leave it to cool a bit and then you

can start consuming it.

Take the remedy on an empty stomach

in the morning before breakfast.

Simple ways of losing weight!

Ingredients:

Ginger root

1.5 liters of water

Lemon

2 tablespoons of apple cider v inegar

Honey

2 tablespoons of apple cider v inegar

Preparation and use:

Prepare warm water, add grated ginger, 2 tablespoonfuls of lemon, and 2 tablespoons of honey. Stir well and drink first thing in the morning and the last thing before you sleep. To prepare ginger water, you will just have to boil the water and add the ginger sliced or grated. Let the mixture simmer for 15 minutes. Remove it from the heat, let it cool, strain it, add a little lemon, and go! Have a glass first thing in the morning and last thing before going to sleep. Try another easy beverage way of

losing weight.

Ingredients

A tablespoon of vinegar

A tablespoon of honey or

ginger One lemon

A bunch of parsley

One cinnamon stick

Preparation and use:

Mix all the ingredients together in

one cup of warm water.

Consume this mixture an hour before

bed preferably with cucumber and

peanut butter. You will soon notice

the results. Enjoy!

Mint, Lemon, and Cucumber-

infused water

Cut half a cucumber into slices, cut

lemons, add organic honey, and a

few mint leaves into warm water.

Keep this in the fridge overnight.

Enjoy this healthy and refreshing

drink during the day!

Almonds

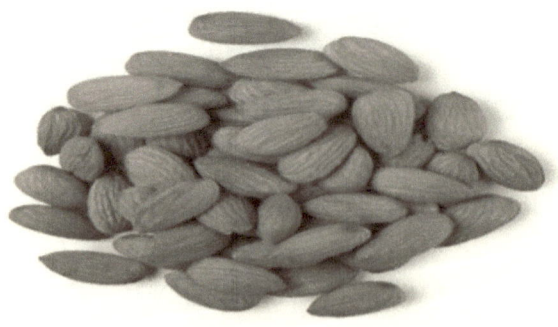

Almonds are among the most health-promoting foods. They prov ide calcium, biotin, iron, magnesium, potassium and omega-fatty acid. Almonds help to reduce blood sugar which helps protect against diabetes and cardiovascular damage. The skin of almonds is rich in flavonoid antioxidants that can prevent coronary heart disease and can reduce risk of cancer. It has no cholesterol, no animal products, and no saturated fats. It is free of gluten and lactose. You can use almond milk for your tea, oatmeal or grits. You can also use it for soup and for baking pastries instead of white flour. Similarly, almond flour can be used as a thickener, sauce or even pudding. You can add grated almonds to your salads and stir-fries. Almond soup is one of my best delicacies. You need to order this soup from me!

Cucumbers

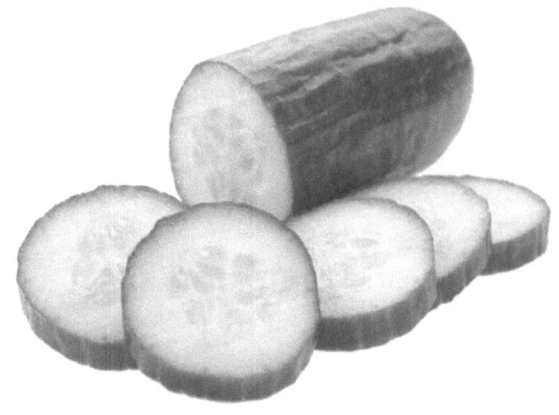

Cucumbers have probably the most neutral taste of all vegetables. They are extremely high in water, low in calories but also have many vital nutrients and plant compounds which can help prevent and treat many health problems. Cucumber is perfect for healthy digestion and can help you lose belly fat. They contain a good amount of soluble fiber. This makes them the ideal food choice for everyone who wants to lose weight and hydrate their body. Cucumbers are high in vitamin C, B and K. They are also rich in potassium, manganese, and copper which help prevents nutrient deficiencies. Their high antioxidant content helps prevent free radical damage associated with aging, heart disease, cancer, lung disease, and autoimmune disease. Add some cucumber to your salad, smoothies, drinks or beverages to get the daily requirement of fiber.

Health Benefits of Cucumbers They...

Fight inflammation

Protect the brain

Protect against cancer

Manage stress

Contain antioxidant properties Improve digestion

Freshen Your Breath

Support Heart Health Maintain a

Healthy Weight

Reduce Blood Glucose

Natural Healing Herbs/Spices

Ginger

Ginger is a famous antioxidant,

popularly used to soothe upset

stomachs. Its strong antioxidant

capabilities make it an excellent

choice in improving your immune

system response. Ginger can be

used fresh, dried, powdered, or as

an oil or juice. Ginger may not have

an immediate impact but may be

effective at reducing the day-to-day progression of muscle pain, joint pain, and stiffness. Ginger has powerful anti-diabetic properties. It can lower blood sugar and improv e heart disease risk factor in patients with type 2 diabetes. Ginger helps alleviate nausea and vomiting. It fights flu and the common cold. Ginger can help treat chronic indigestion because it speeds up the emptying of the stomach. It can also help reduce menstrual pain or dysmenorrhea--which refers to pain felt during a woman's menstrual cycle-- when taken at the beginning of the menstrual period. It is used as an

ingredient in laxatives, anti-gas,

and antacid medications.

Research shows that ginger can

protect against age-related damage

to the brain. It can also improv e brain

function in elderly women. Chewing

raw ginger or drinking ginger tea is a

common home remedy for nausea

during cancer treatment because of

the presence of a powerful compound

called 6-gingerol. Ginger fights fungal

infections and it helps kill off disease-

causing fungi due to its

powerful anti-fungal properties. Ginger can be used to make stew, soups and stir-fries. It can be chopped or crushed and used in curries and savory dishes.

It can also be used in drinks and beverages. That is why this spice belongs in every kitchen.

Here are some tasty ways to use ginger: Add fresh ginger to a smoothie or juice Add fresh or dried ginger to a stir-fry or homemade salad dressing Make ginger tea by putting steep peeled fresh ginger in boiling water Use fresh or dried ginger to spice up any fish recipe

Turmeric

Turmeric or Curcuma longa as it is called scientifically has significant immunostimulant abilities. A golden spice, when added with black pepper, it absorbs more effectively. Curcumin in turmeric and piperine in black pepper have been shown to improv e health due to their anti-inflammatory, antioxidant and disease-fighting qualities.

This can help:

Decrease inflammation,

Better digestion

Aid weight loss

Fight cancer

Reduce pain and arthritis.

You can add it to your stir fry, fried

eggs, sauce, or use it to make tea.

Ginseng

Ginseng is known for its powerful

antioxidant abilities. It can help lower

blood sugar and help treat diabetes.

Ginseng is known to be able to boost

immunity. It particularly strengthens the

immune system in people with cancer.

Ginseng is often used to reduce

inflammation. It could help improv e or

treat erectile dysfunction. Ginseng may

help to increase energy and can

help to stimulate physical and mental activity in people who feel weak and tired.

Garlic

Eating garlic is regarded as a great way to fight heart disease and keep your blood vessels clear from blockage. Eating garlic may help to regulate blood sugar levels, as well as stop or decrease the effects of some diabetes complications. It also fights infections and reduces cholesterol.

Cinnamon

Cinnamon is an excellent source of fiber and the trace mineral manganese is a very good source of calcium. It can help improv e glucose. Cinnamon oil also has very powerful antibiotic, antiseptic, and analgesic benefits. It helps in preventing and giving relief from anxiety, tension, and memory loss. It helps in strengthening and improving your brain activity. When you use cinnamon oil regularly, it will help in the following:

• maintenance of normal blood sugar levels.

• Improving your metabolic activity

• Reducing blood pressure

• Helps in supporting healthier digestion

• Easing the removal of waste from the body

• Reducing bloating.

• Reducing the risk of heart attack and stroke

Celery

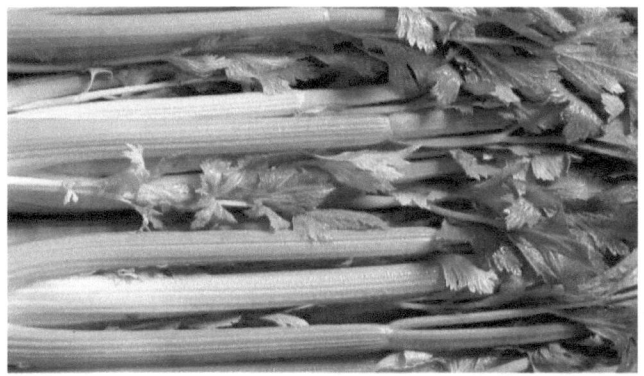

Celery, which is one of my favorite superfoods, is an excellent source of calcium, vitamins, and fiber. It boosts digestion, relieves bloating, and lowers blood pressure and high cholesterol. It also prevents cancer by improving on detoxification. You can add celery to your diet to help protect and improv e heart health. Celery seed extracts can treat high blood pressure because of their anti-hypertensive properties. Celery is loaded with potassium and calcium. Celery is an ideal liver cleansing food. It can help protect kidney health and prevent liver diseases. It contains diuretic properties. Celery can remove toxins, wastes, and contaminants from your body. Celery can aid in weight loss because it's low in calories. Celery also provides essential minerals, vitamins, and vital nutrients. It boosts lipid metabolism and is rich in electrolytes, antioxidants, potassium, Iron, vitamin B and vitamin C. It can be eaten with peanut butter, added to your salads, stir-fries, sauces, and soup. You can make celery juice easily. Buy organic celery, rinse the celery and run it through a juicer or you can chop the celery and blend it in a high-speed blender until it is smooth. Strain well and drink immediately.

Black Pepper

Black pepper is one of the most common spices added to cuisines around the world. Its spiciness is due to the chemical compound known as piperine. It contains antioxidant and anti-inflammatory properties. Black pepper can help the metabolic breakdown of turmeric compounds in the stomach and the liver. Black pepper aids in weight loss, and helps in relieving sinus, asthma, and nasal congestion. It also reduces the risk of cancer, and heart and liver ailments. It has antioxidants that can prevent or repair the damage caused by free radicals and help prevent many diseases. As black pepper is carminative in nature, it easily expels gas out of the body. Peppery foods are a good way to help you shed weight naturally. Black pepper can be added to tonics or warm water for treating cold and cough. It also prov ides relief from sinusitis and nasal congestion. It has an expectorant property that helps break up the mucus and phlegm depositions in the respiratory tract. Black pepper has the antibacterial property that can help fight against infections and insect bites. It helps reduce memory impairment and cognitive malfunction because of its piperine. Piperine is an alkaloid. This is the thing that gives black pepper a lot of its qualities, like its noticeable spiciness and its pungent taste. Piperine is effective at combating free radical damage or oxidative stress in and around your cells. They help you fight premature aging, cell death, and poor cell function. Piperine can lower blood glucose levels. Pepper is a strong spice that contains antibiotic and healing properties. It can be used for treating strep throat.

Rosemary

This spice contains active ingredients that can protect the brain from free radical damage and other negative influences that can affect your memory. Rosemary essential oil is highly effective in improving memory and helping you study better. It can also help reduce pain as well as lower cortisol.

Probiotics and Prebiotics: Knowing the Difference!

Even though probiotics and prebiotics sound similar, the two plays different roles for your health. Probiotics are important and beneficial bacteria while prebiotics is food for these bacteria. Probiotics are liv e bacteria found in certain foods or supplements. They can prov ide numerous health benefits. While prebiotics are substances that come from certain types of carbs (mostly fiber) that humans can't digest. Eating balanced amounts of both pro- and prebiotics will make you have the right balance of these bacteria that will improve your overall health. Probiotics are beneficial bacteria found in certain foods or supplements. Prebiotics are types of fiber that feed the friendly bacteria in the digestive system. The good bacteria in your digestive tract help protect you from harmful bacteria and fungi. They also send signals to your immune system and help regulate inflammation. Some of your stomach bacteria form vitamin K and short-chain fatty acids. Short-chain fatty acids are the main nutrient source of the cells lining the colon. They promote a strong stomach barrier that helps keep out harmful substances, viruses, and bacteria. This also reduces inflammation and may reduce the risk of cancer. Prebiotics are types of fiber found in vegetables, fruits, and legumes. These types of fiber are not digestible by humans, but your good stomach bacteria can digest them. Foods that are high in prebiotic fiber include legumes, beans and peas, oats, bananas, berries, asparagus, dandelion greens, garlic, leeks, and onions. These types of fiber prov ide nutrients to the bacteria that support healthy digestion and immune function. There are many probiotic foods that naturally contain helpful bacteria, such as yogurt. A high-quality, plain yogurt with liv e cultures can be a fantastic addition to your diet if you want to add beneficial bacteria. Fermented foods are another great option, as they contain beneficial bacteria that thrive on the naturally occurring sugar or fiber in the food. Examples of fermented foods are Sauerkraut, kimchi, kombucha tea, kefir (dairy and non-dairy), pickles (non-pasteurized). A good time to take your probiotics is after you eat, and it's best to take your probiotics alongside a meal. Food can provide your probiotic with the proper nourishment it needs to survive, grow, and multiply once in your

stomach. You can get your prebiotics

and probiotics from any retail store. I

usually get my supplements from Vitamin

World. They usually have

varieties and are budget friendly

because of their generosity with

coupons. They did not pay me to

advertise but I just prefer to buy from

them because they sav e me some

money even after buying all my

vitamins, herbal teas, and

other nutritional supplements.

The Brain Foods

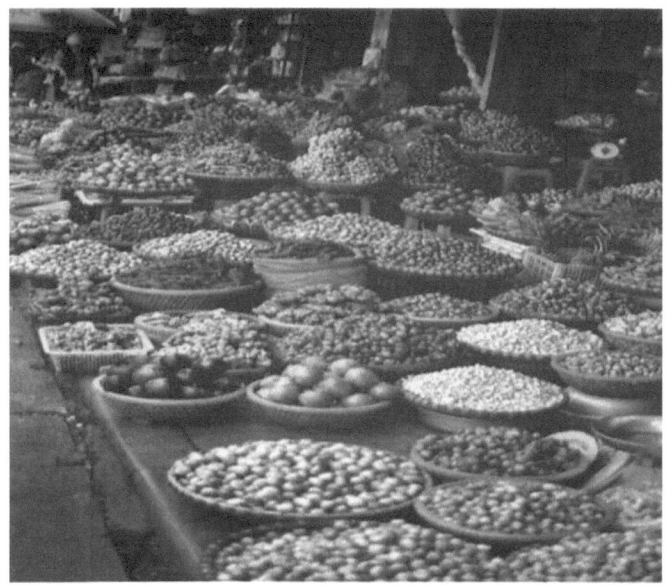

Nuts

Almonds, walnuts, pistachios can

strengthen brain function. They have

antioxidants that have been linked to

lower cholesterol and lower risk of

cardiovascular disease. They can also

reduce stress-induced blood pressure. Ironically, most people may be surprised that the perfect brain food is reading because it gives insight and a better understanding of things. My love for books is one of my secret weapons. Knowledge is power!

Apple Cider Vinegar

Apple cider vinegar is made by a slow fermentation process, leaving it rich in bioactive components. It is useful for health purposes, cleaning, and hygiene. "Mother" of vinegar is the cobweb-like amino acid-based substance found in unprocessed, unfiltered vinegar, which shows it's the best quality. It contains potassium and enzymes to help banish fatigue.

Benefits of Apple Cider Vinegar

Apple Cider Vinegar has been used as a home remedy for many things. It is one of the best natural treatments for many diseases. It has natural antiviral and anti-bacterial properties. It has alkaline abilities, contains lots of minerals, can lower both your cholesterol and blood pressure, and even regulate your blood sugar levels. It's also good for restoring the good bacteria in your stomach, as well as giving your immune system a well-needed boost. Apple cider Vinegar also helps to:

• Increase Resting Metabolism More Than 130%

• Flush out harmful toxins

• Boost energy levels and improve

• Block excess fat production

• Support the heart and other organs

• Build strong bones and teeth

• Soothe and heal chronic skin conditions—even smooth out wrinkles

• Ease nausea, improv e digestion, and control weight

- Relieve nerve and joint pain

- Flush out toxins and boost immunity

Mix 1-2 teaspoons of organic

Apple Cider Vinegar with a glass

of warm water.

Ingredients for treating a Sinus infection

Half a cup of water

One tablespoon of raw honey

One tablespoon of cayenne pepper

A quarter cup of Apple cider vinegar

One lemon juice

How to prepare this remedy?

Bring the water to boil. Take a glass and

make a mixture of the water and the

Apple cider vinegar. To this mixture,

add honey and cayenne pepper, and make sure to stir well. Finally, add the lemon juice. Consume this beverage on a regular basis until you feel better.

Recipe for Sore Throat

Gargle with a mixture of about one-third cup of apple cider vinegar mixed with warm water as needed. Brew up a cup tea and sweetened with honey. This can help soothe your sore throat.

CHAPTER 4

Fuel up on Superfoods

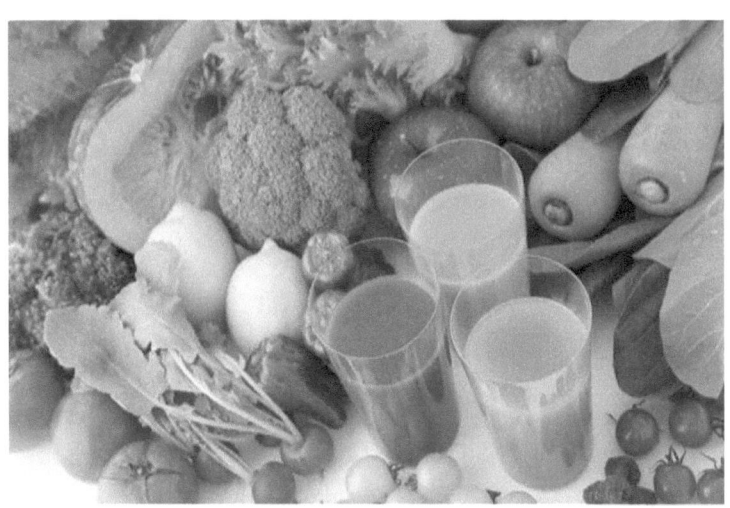

Superfoods work wonders for your immune system. They are also good for organ health and weight loss. These superfoods will:

- Build your immune system

- Lower the risk of heart disease

- Balance cholesterol

- Eliminate headaches

- Give energy and strength

- Reverse diabetes

- Eliminate cancer cells

- Reduce weight

- Curb hunger and sugar cravings

Superfoods include kale, brussels sprouts, lemon, cherries, blueberries, and mushrooms. Mushrooms are high in fiber, potassium, vitamin C, selenium and vitamin D. Kale is high in vitamin K, vitamin A, vitamin C and powerful antioxidants, which help protect against some cancers.

Spirulina is a green-blue-algae superfood that is a plant-based protein with great health benefits. Spirulina is high in fatty acids, full of vitamins, and very nutritious. It has a cleansing and detox property that can assist in waste elimination. It boosts the immune system, improv es digestion, and normalizes blood pressure. Most Olympic athletes have used it for stamina and improv ed performance. It helps with Alzheimer's and Parkinson's diseases. It also helps remove toxins in the body as well as promote healthy bacteria flora in the intestine. It can help alleviate sinus issues. It can help to reduce cholesterol and lower the chance of stroke. Add a tablespoon to your water, yogurt, and tea.

Chlorella is another plant-based green algae superfood that can help improve digestion, prevent cancer, heart disease, normalize blood pressure, lower blood sugar, and boost the immune system. It also helps in detoxifying toxins in the body.

Ashwagandha

Ashwagandha is a plant which root

and berry are used to make medicines.

It is popularly known as Indian Ginseng.

It helps to relieve stress and anxiety. It

also decreases depression.

Ashwagandha is used to reduce level

of fat and sugar in the blood.

According to Sharwa (1999), "The root

of Ashwagandha is regarded as tonic,

aphrodisiac, narcotic, diuretic,

anthelmintic, astringent, thermogenic

and stimulant. The root smells like horse

("ashwa"), that is why it is called

Ashwagandha (on consuming it gives

the power of a horse). It is commonly

used in treating emaciation in children

(when given with milk, it is the best

tonic for children), debility from old

age, rheumatism, constipation,

insomnia, nervous breakdown, goiter

etc. It also acts as a stimulant and

increases sperm count. Ashwagandha

when used in the treatment of fibroid

tumors of the uterus showed reduction

of uterine bleeding tendencies and

disappearance of fibroids after long

treatment (Abbas et al. 2004, 2005).

Beets

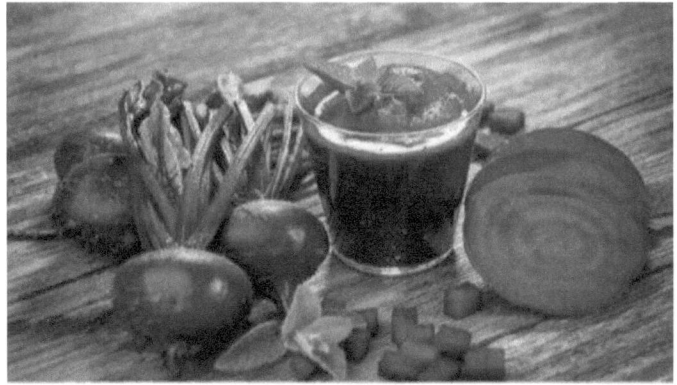

Beets are loaded with antioxidants and have been found to protect against cancer, heart disease, and inflammation. It will boost your stamina. Beets are naturally sweet and full of fiber, iron, calcium, and vitamin C. They are anticancer and have a lot of health-promoting properties. Beet juice can help lower blood pressure within hours. Beets can detoxify the system and boost blood flow in the brain. Beets are highly recommended for improving the mental performance of a person.

Pomegranate

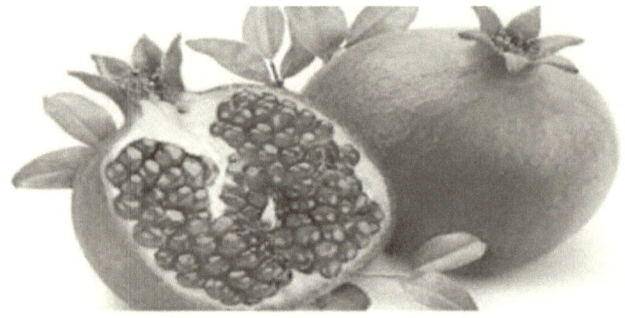

Pomegranate is rich in antioxidants and helps in improving heart disease and cardiovascular disease. This is an antiviral, antimicrobial and antioxidant. It is very delicious. You can add it to

your soup especially okra soup

which will lower your blood sugar.

Cranberries

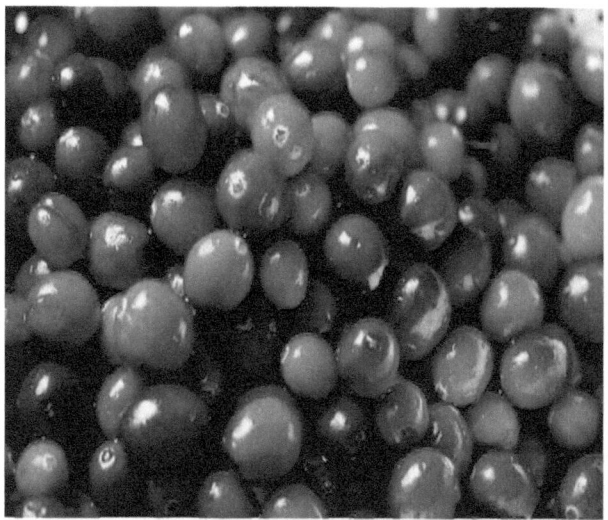

Cranberries are renowned for

protecting against urinary tract

infections. They may improv e blood

cholesterol and aid in recovery from

strokes. Cranberry juice has also been

shown to make cancer drugs more

potent. It helps prevent kidney stones and treats bladder infection. Cranberry water can balance Ph to suppress your hunger. It can as well destroy stubborn cellulites and detoxify your liver.

Flaxseed

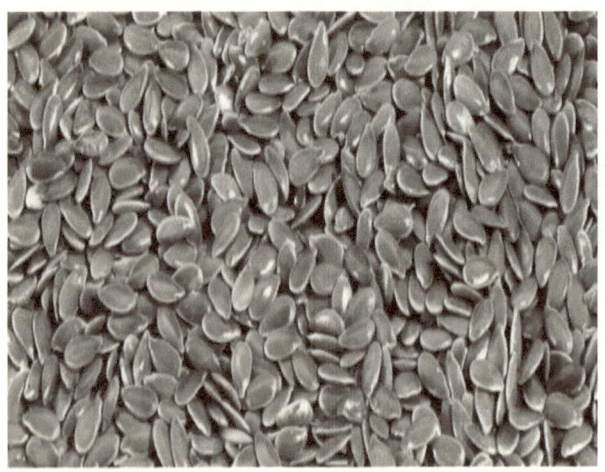

Flaxseed lowers blood cholesterol, which is a fatty compound you can find in most tissues in your body as well as in your bloodstream. It helps your

body digest different foods and

encourages hormone production.

Flaxseed reduces the risk of heart

attack, but it is also a rich source of

lignan, a powerful antioxidant that

may be a powerful ally against

disease and certain cancers,

especially breast cancer.

Quinoa

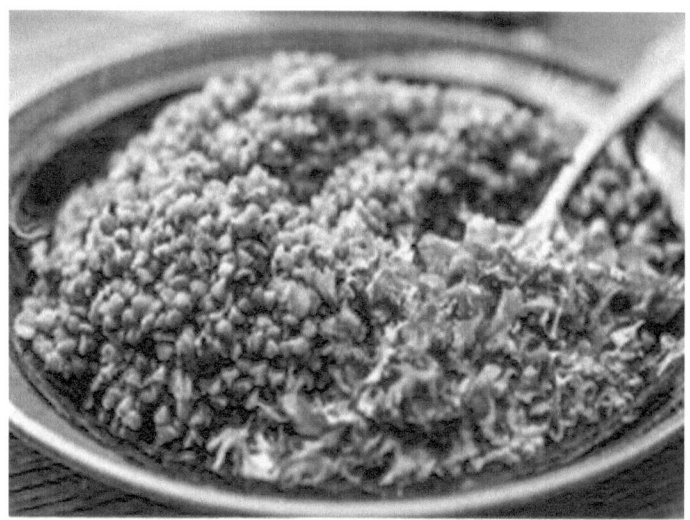

Packed with a variety of nutrients, including iron and copper, it is gluten-free and high in fiber. This ancient seed is known as "the mother of all grains." Quinoa contains all the essential amino acids, making it a complete protein good for vegans and vegetarians. It is also a great source of magnesium, which relaxes blood vessels and has been found to reduce the frequency of migraines. Quinoa is a super seed which is prepared like a grain. It is an amino acid-rich protein seed. It is best eaten with seafood dishes and mixes well with beans. It helps you get energy

from the food you eat thereby

maintaining your red blood cells.

Researchers have found that it

reduces the risk of high blood

pressure and heart attack.

Raspberries

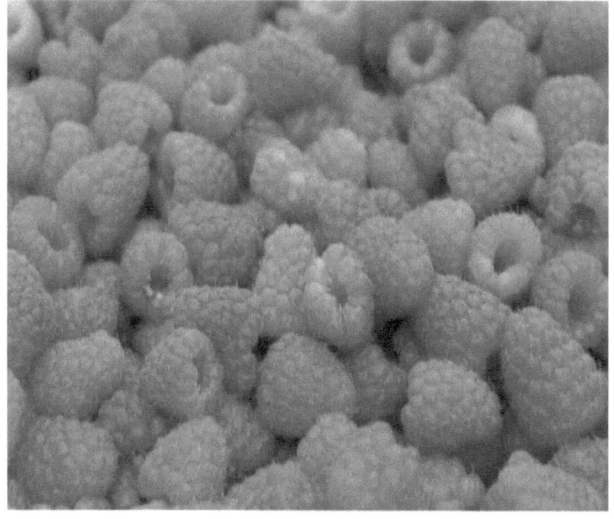

This berry is tart, sweet, and incredibly

juicy. Berries prov ide fiber, vitamin C,

and manganese. Raspberries also

contain a powerful arsenal

of antioxidants.

Spinach

Powerful antioxidants in spinach have

been found to combat a variety of

cancers, including ovarian, breast, and

colon cancers. It's good for your brain.

Research indicates that spinach

reduces the decline in brain function

associated with aging and protects the

heart from cardiovascular disease.

Although it contains relatively high

amounts of iron and calcium, oxalate

compounds bind to these minerals and

diminish their absorption.

Walnuts

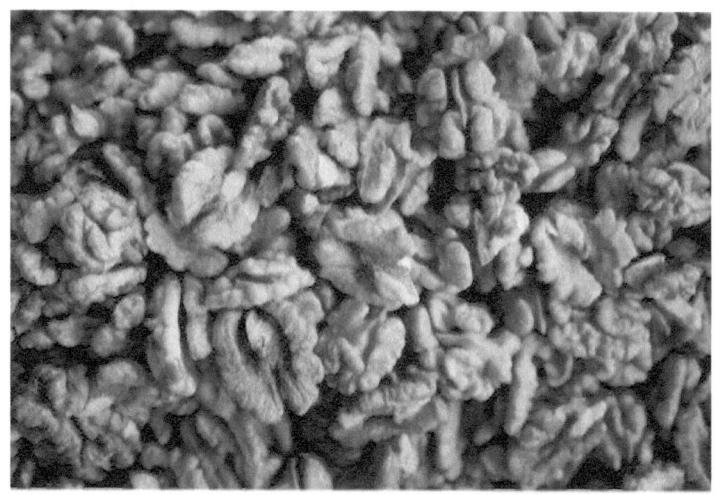

Walnut is probably the best food for the brain. It contains plenty of vitamin C, K, and antioxidants. Walnut supplies omega-3 fatty acids which aid in everything from maintaining cognitive function, to improving cholesterol and blood pressure. Toss a few toasted walnut halves on your oatmeal, another heart-healthy superfood or try them on your favorite salad for a tasty crunch. Add walnut to your smoothie.

Acai

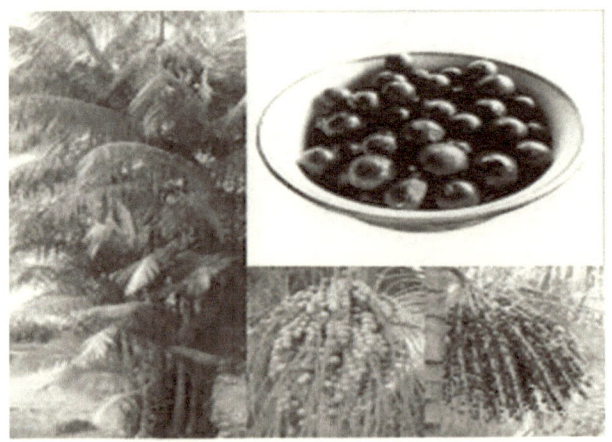

This is an American palm tree producing small edible blackish-purple berries. Acai is a powerful antioxidant with a low-sugar fruit lev el and heart-healthy fats. It helps keep your sugar lev el low and promotes longevity.

Banana

Bananas can help improv e your mood and blood pressure. It is packed full of potassium which is one of the electrolytes. A banana has about 30% of your daily recommended intake of vitamin B6. Vitamin B6 helps the brain produce serotonin, which can help stabilize your mood. Bananas help you sleep and digest food. It also helps relieve depression and anxiety by stimulating the serotonin lev el in your body. Bananas protect against heart disease and stroke. However, if you don't eat bananas often like me, you

can add it to your recipe to make

a delicious smoothie.

Avocado

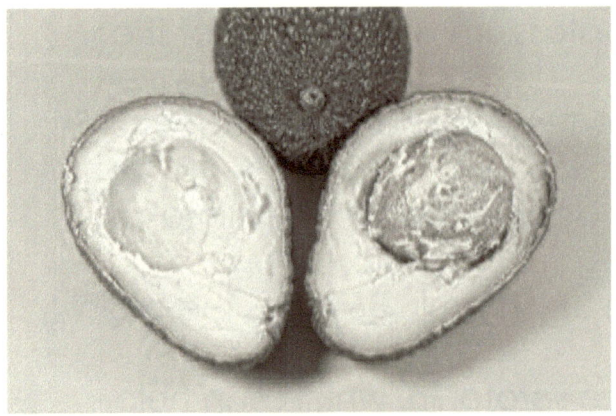

This is one of the healthiest fruits you

can eat. They are rich in

monosaturated fat that help to keep

you full and satiated. Avocado has

lutein which is very good for your eyes.

It can boost cognitive function,

memory, and concentration.

Watercress

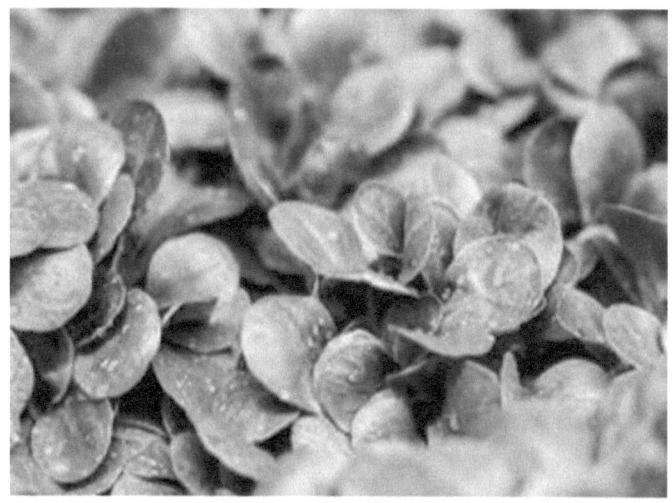

Research shows that just 1 cup of watercress supplies nearly 100% of a woman's recommended daily amount of vitamin K, which has been shown to prevent hardening of the arteries and is essential for strong bones. It is also a good source of folic acid and vitamin A, a potent antioxidant. It supplies iron which helps in the prevention of anemia. Try these peppery leaves in salads, sandwiches, or toss them in a quick stir-fry or soup.

Chia Seeds

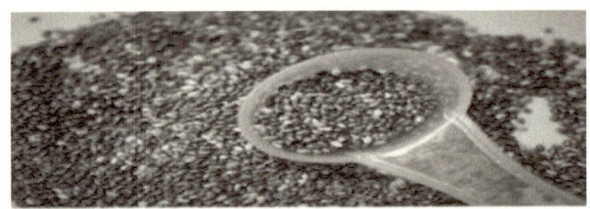

These tiny seeds are rich in omega-3 fatty acid and high in fiber, protein, and minerals. They are plant-based calcium and a major hunger buster. They are low in calories and aid digestion. You can add chia seeds to your oats, salads, coconut water or yogurt.

Coconut

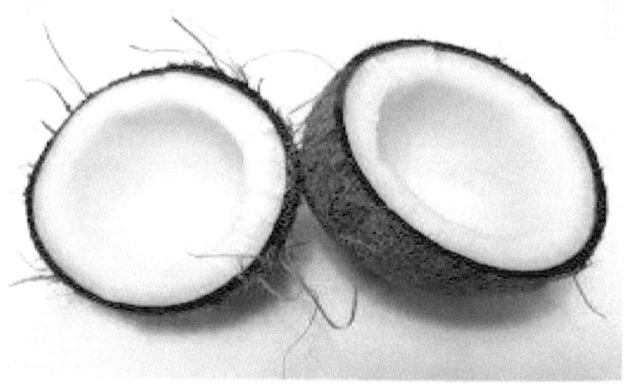

Coconut is a superfood and one of the miracle drinks which has wide and diverse benefits. It can be used for skin care or hair care. It lowers blood pressure, and cholesterol levels. Coconut oil is antifungal and supports a healthy stomach. It is used for reducing inflammation and treating age-related memory loss.

Coconut milk is antimicrobial and antiviral. It is rich in potassium and contains heart-healthy fat.

Apples

Apples are the richest fruit source of pectin, a soluble fiber that has been shown to lower blood pressure, reduce cholesterol, decrease the risk of colon and breast cancers, asthma, and maybe even lessen the severity of diabetes. "An apple a day keeps the doctor away" – the old saying goes. Apples are a good source of vitamins and minerals. It is great when you mix

apples with other fruits to make

healthy fruit salads.

SUPERFOOD DRINKS

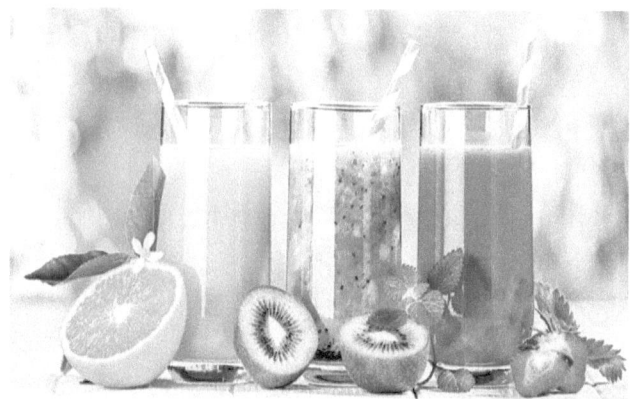

These drinks are for detox, cleansing,

building the immune system and giving

you nutritional benefits for a life full of

health and wellness. These drinks are full

of vitamins which modern-day drinks

lack and the few that contain these

vitamins are expensive. The vitamins

contain antibacterial, antifungal, and antiviral properties. Vitamin C has anti-inflammatory properties. The Proteins are great for meal replacement and do contain little or no sugar.

The healthy drinks are high in fiber with low calories. The drink helps flush harmful toxins out of your body. Natural juice is very beneficial because it:

• Improv es energy

• Has great taste

• Improv es nutritional quality

•   • increases the intake of health-promoting phytochemicals

•   • It's fun and enjoyable

Flat belly juice

1 grapefruit

1 tablespoon of honey

2 tablespoons of apple cider

vinegar A small piece of ginger

8 oz of warm water

Blend together and enjoy your

drink any time of the day!

Belly Flat beverage

1 cucumber

I lemon

10 pieces of mint leaves

A small piece of ginger

32 oz of water Cut the ingredient in

pieces into a jar. Allow to soak for few

hours. Drink throughout day and

enjoy yourself!

Hot lemon tea

Lemon

Ginger

Cinnamon

2 tablespoons of apple cider

2 tablespoons of honey

Bring to a boil, lemon, grated

ginger, and cinnamon.

Sieve into a cup, add 2 tablespoon of

honey and 2 tablespoon of apple

cider vinegar. Stir and enjoy!

Smoothies

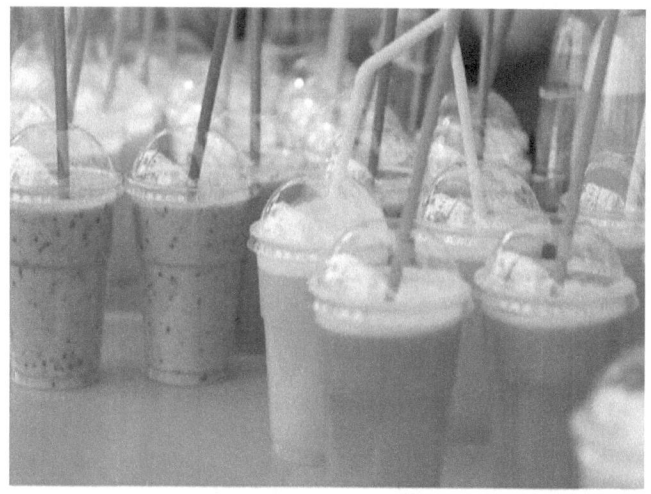

These are fresh fruits with plenty of vitamins and minerals. They are also full of fiber and very nutritious. It is the easiest, quickest, and fastest way to eat healthy because you can blend anything into a smoothie. To make a smoothie you need your fresh fruits (which is your base), liquids, and ice.

Just be determined and buy a good blender like Vitamix.

High-performance smoothie

I lemon 1 banana

1 cup of ice

I cup of coconut water/ almond milk

Blend together until smooth and enjoy!

Night Food/Snacks

Eat proteins such as an omelet with vegetables, avocado, flaxseed, chicken. Cucumber is extremely good to eat at night if you really want to lose belly fat. Drink yogurt. Leafy greens such as kale, spinach, collards, swiss chards with salmon or tuna.

The Cheat Days

Most of us have our cheat days because we may not strictly follow our health or weight loss plan and we may overeat during parties, job orientations, or holidays. However, we are supposed to liv e and enjoy life to the full. Occasionally, we may dine at a restaurant or attend a party where we may eat food to curb our cravings. Make it a habit to eat slowly, so you can enjoy the food. Eating slowly also aids in digestion. Drink plenty of water to flush your system. You can also drink apple cider vinegar mixed with lemon and warm water. This works well to

detox and cleanse your system.

Exercise is vital to good health and it

enhances detoxification. Two days of a

healthy meal is equivalent to three

days of going to the gym. Nonetheless,

eating a healthy meal and going to the

gym are powerful assets to cultivate.

You must be your own cheerleader and

supporter. Love yourself!

CHAPTER 5

DIABETES

This is excessive sugar in a person's body. Lifestyle changes influence blood glucose level. Mediterranean diets and low-fat vegetarian diets may be the best food for diabetes patients because they are based on legumes, whole grains, fruits, vitamins, and proteins. The Mediterranean diet uses olive oil which is very good for the heart. However, try to eat whole foods and plant-based foods like vegetables, whole grains, salmon, and beans. Monitor your blood sugar daily. Eating smaller portions of food are great. I learned from my research that any food label ingredient that ends with the letters 'ose' is sugar such as fructose, galactose, sucrose, lactose. Monitor your A1c, which is known as Hemoglobin A1c. This is the standard for measuring the quantity of blood sugar in people with diabetes. It is advisable that your A1C should be about 7 percent.

Get Enough Sleep

Getting good quality sleep is essential for good health. I never knew that poor sleep and lack of rest can impact your insulin sensitivity and blood glucose levels. Also, lack of sleep can increase your appetite and even lead to weight gain. I have learned from experience that it is not only sugar intake that causes diabetes but also stress can lead to your sugar becoming elevated likewise the lack of sleep. Sleep deprivation increases sugar cravings and chronic stress increases the production of cortisol which causes an increase in blood sugar, cholesterol, and belly fat. I have learned that getting enough quality sleep is important in the treatment of

diabetes, blood pressure, and heart

disease. **Regulate Your Blood Sugar**

* Change your diet: Eat a low-

processed, anti-Inflammatory diet.

You can regulate your blood sugar by

avoiding sugar and carbohydrates

like white bread, white rice or cake.

Eat a good amount of proteins, fiber

and healthy fats in all your meals.

* Exercise: walking, jogging, swimming,

and other physical exercises help cells

in your muscles to take up more

glucose in order to use it for energy and

tissue repair. It also makes cells

more responsive to insulin and

helps prevent resistance.

* Sleep: a lack of sleep can raise

stress and appetite hormones.

Have an 8-hour sleep pattern.

*Healthy fats such as coconut oil, MCT

oil (Medium-chain triglyceride), extra

virgin olive oil, nuts, and seeds (like

almonds, Chia, hemp, and flax), and

avocado. Coconut oil, ghee, and

grass-fed butter.

Take probiotic and digestive enzymes

to help break down your food and put

healthy bacteria in your stomach in

order to reduce inflammation.

Herbs/Food to Lower Blood Sugar

These foods can improv e your overall health and make you say goodbye to diabetes. The more fiber you eat, the fuller you become. I tried it and it worked for me. Studies indicate that taking this herb can help lower hemoglobin and fasting blood glucose levels in people with type 2 diabetes.

Holy Basil – Hot Basil: According to study the extracts from holy basil might help reduce postprandial and fasting blood sugar in people who have type 2 diabetes. It contains powerful antioxidants which can prevent damage to your cell and organs. It can help to produce insulin due to beta cells functions in your pancreas.

Yogurt: Probiotic yogurt is a fermented food which contains plenty of vitamin D, protein, and calcium. It lowers blood glucose level and lowers systolic blood pressure.

Ginger: The benefit of consuming ginger is great. It can reduce body weight and reduces body fat mass. Ginger can raise the levels of insulin as well as decrease blood sugar lev els. It's an anti-nausea aide and aids digestion. It helps to reduce pain like menstruation pain and osteoarthritis pain.

Garlic: This herb is used for many therapeutic purposes despite the odor. Garlic fights viruses, fungus, and bacteria. It helps prevent sugar spikes. Adding raw garlic to your vegetables, fish, or meat will intensify the flavor and deliver good health benefits.

Cinnamon: Cinnamon can lower blood sugar and cholesterol in people who have type 2 diabetes. A small amount of cinnamon might have great influence. It is very cost effective to buy stick cinnamon in bulk since it has a longer shelf life.

Barley: A good source of copper, vitamin B1, chromium, phosphorus, magnesium, and niacin. Barley can help to steady blood sugar levels and lower high cholesterol.

Bitter Leaf: A bitter plant whose leaves, extracts, stems and barks are used for culinary, medicinal and curative purposes. Bitter leaf contains Vitamin A, Vitamin C, Vitamin E, Vit.B1 and Vit.B2. It helps to reduce high sugar lev el in the blood. It can help alleviate mild stomach ailments. It also speeds up metabolism and is great for weight loss. It is used preparing the popular African bitter leaf soup.

Bitter kola: This is also known as Garcia kola. It has antibacterial, detoxification, and cleansing properties. Bitter kola contains chemical compounds that will help the breakdown of glycogen in the liver. A natural hunger suppressant and you will increase the urge to drink more water.

American Ginseng: According to research, American ginseng can lower blood sugar levels in people who have type 2 diabetes. This may be due to the stimulation of insulin release and tissue insulin sensitization.

Aloe Vera: Aloe Vera is part of the Lily plant family. It contains protein, calcium, magnesium, and vitamin A and E. Aloe Vera has around 240 species, but only 4 have nutritional value. According to research, the gel from Aloe Vera might lower blood sugar level. It is also used to ease constipation and digestive systems.

Blueberries: Blueberries are lower when it comes to naturally occurring sugars. This is in comparison to other fruits.

Research shows that the bioactive compounds in blueberries increase the sensiti ity to insulin.

Avocado: The monounsaturated, healthy fat found in avocados slows the release of sugar into the bloodstreams.

Okra: Ground okra seeds and peels help reduce blood sugar levels. You can successfully reduce your blood glucose after drinking okra water in the morning. Okra is high in fiber. It aids in digestion, cuts hunger cravings, and keeps those who eat it fuller for longer. Drinking "okra water" is a popular new method of using okra. The drink is made by putting okra pods in water and soaking them overnight. The nutrients in the skin and seed pods will be absorbed into the water.

Salmon is a great source of omega-3 fatty acid that improv es insulin resistance. A study shows 8 ounces of seafood a week reduces heart-related diseases.

Oats: It lowers bad LDL cholesterol and improves insulin resistance. Oatmeal is rich in antioxidants.

Lentils: This legume is high in fiber and protein. It can keep you fuller and lowers the risk of heart disease.

Grapefruit: This fruit contains many flavonoids. It can help lowers blood sugar and cholesterol. It has cancer-fighting compounds as well as help prevents liver damage.

Bitter melon: Contains many nutrients that can be beneficial to your health. It's linked to lowering blood sugar, which some studies suggest means it can aid in diabetes treatment especially type 2 diabetes. It contains an insulin-like compound known as polypeptide-p or vegetable insulin. It is said to contain antiviral protein. As an antioxidant, the fruit can lower bad cholesterol levels, which can reduce the risk of getting heart disease. Bitter melon aids in digestion, relieves bloating, upset stomach, occasional nausea and heartburn, as well as supports the liver function and healthy skin.

Diabetes Meal Plan

This is a guide on the kinds of food to eat and how much to consume at snack and at meal time. The key to a healthy diet is to choose the right portion sizes and to include a variety of different healthy foods. Choose foods that prov ide the highest quality nutrients of its food group. To be more accurate, choose foods that are rich in fiber, minerals, and vitamins. ***Think of Your Plate as a Clock***

The best thing you can do is imagine your plate is a clock. Half of your plate should be fruits and vegetables. A quarter should be lean protein, such as beans, baked fish, and chicken. The last quarter should be reserved for (preferably whole) grains. Go for foods with low GI. The GI, i.e., glycemic index was designed in order to estimate the blood glucose response of the body to foods which have carbs.

Marvelous morning drink

½ lemon

I tablespoon of honey

1 teaspoon of apple cider vinegar in

a cup.

Warm water

This will boast your energy lev el for

the day.

Cinnamon drink

Organic cloves – 3 g

Organic cinnamon –

2 sticks

Warm water

Add the ingredients in water, let them soak about 3 minutes, strain the mixture and enjoy!

Okra drink

3 Okra

1 qt (32 FL oz) warm water

Cut okra in pieces into a warm water and soaked overnight.

Drink first thing in the morning. It will lower your glucose level. You will feel full and good through the day. Enjoy it!

Recipe for Cold and Flu:

Ingredients

1 large knob of ginger

2 Cinnamon sticks

4 cups of water

1 lemon

2 tablespoons of organic honey

2 tablespoons of apple cider vinegar

Bring to boil the grated ginger, cinnamon, and sliced lemon. Strain in a container.

Add the 2 tablespoons of organic honey and 2 tablespoons of apple cider vinegar. Enjoy!

Energy smoothie

Recipe and ingredients:

5 bananas

2 kiwis Handful

of kale

2 apples

How to prepare:

Put the ingredients in a blender and blend the combination fast so that you get a smooth paste.

Add half a liter of water to this dose.

Drink half of the combination in the morning while drinking the rest of it throughout the day.

Enrich this drink with great amounts of veggies, fruits, and Salmon. Enjoy!

Recipe for Grated Sweet Potato and Zucchini Bread

Ingredients:

Dried rosemary – 1 tablespoon

One finely chopped onion

Two crushed garlic cloves

Baking soda – 1 teaspoon

Grated zucchini – 450 grams or 2 cups peeled and grated sweet potato – 250 grams

1 cup black pepper and sea salt

Almond meal – 150 grams or one cup Cherry tomatoes

Five lightly beaten eggs

– ¼ cup Organic cheese or nutritional yeast. First, preheat the oven to 200°C or 400°F and take a baking dish and line it with parchment paper.

In a big bowl mix sweet potato, organic cheese or nutritional yeast, zucchini, rosemary, pepper, salt, and almonds. Mix well all ingredients, then add the 5 eggs and mix once more. Bake for 40 to 50 minutes. Your bread is ready when you insert a skewer and the skewer comes out clean.

Make Your Kitchen Heavenly

When you edit your fridge, and you have all the wonderful plant-based foods in your kitchen, it makes your kitchen heavenly. In as much as it's essential to av oid some foods like junk food, I have realized that what you don't eat will cause you to be sick, fatigued, stressed, and have low mental clarity. I determined to use the best oil in my kitchen such as olive oil, coconut oil, avocado oil, grape seed oil, flaxseed oil, almond oil, and palm oil. Though these best oils are more expensive compared to other not-so-healthy oils, the benefit to your health makes them worth the price. I usually visit Vitamin World for varieties of wellness supplements and herbs. Vitamin World always offers buy 1, get 1 free mix & match on Vitamin World & precision engineered brand items aside coupons and discounts. As a prudent woman, I like discounts and coupons, it sav es me a lot of money. Also, I highly recommend that you take your vitamin supplements. It will make your health awesome.

PRAYER

I pray that God will give you the wisdom, understanding, strength of character and discipline to apply the knowledge you have gained in this book to transform your life. I pray that you will be enjoy good health and fulfil God's purpose for your life in Jesus name. Amen.

Contact me via:

www.cphealthyliving.com

cphealthyliving@gmail.com

ebonychi@yahoo.com

Women of Asset face book page

References

Nelson, Miriam E., and Judy Knipe. Strong Women Eat Well: Nutritional Strategies for a Healthy Body and Mind. Perigee, 2005.

Ramsey, D. (2013). The total money makeover: A proven plan for financial fitness (Classic ed.). Nashville, TN: Thomas Nelson.

Sharma GS. Ashwagandharishta - Rastantra Sar Evam Sidhyaprayog Sangrah - Krishna-Gopal Ayurveda Bhawan (Dharmarth Trust) Nagpur: 1938. pp. 743–744.

Singh RS. Ashwagandha, Vanaushadhi

Nidharsika (Ayurvedic Pharmacopia)

UP Sansthan: 1983. pp. 30–31.

WIDERSTROM, JEN. DIET RIGHT

FOR YOUR PERSONALITY TYPE:

The Revolutionary

Week Weight-Loss Plan That ... Works

for You. HARMONY CROWN, 2018.

www.ingramcontent.com/pod-product-compliance
Lightning Source LLC
Chambersburg PA
CBHW021548290526
45784CB00016B/837